Eleven Life Lessons for Teenagers
(and Everyone Else)

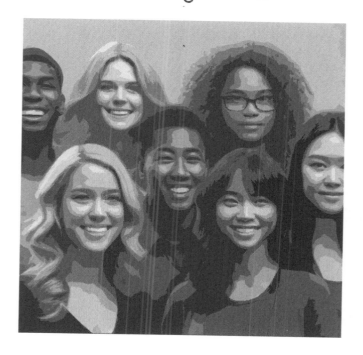

by Michael Lisagor

D1707032

Printed in the United States of America

10 9 8 7 6 5 4 3 2 1

Library of Congress Cataloging-in-Publication Data

Eleven Lessons for Teenagers (and Everyone Else)

ISBN: 9798321164884

Teen & Young Adult: Personal Health, Depression & Mental Health

"Words spoken from the heart have the power to change a person's life. They can even melt the icy walls of mistrust that separate peoples and nations."

- Daisaku Ikeda

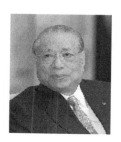

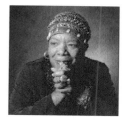

"I've learned that people will forget what you said, people will forget what you did, but people will never forget how you made them feel."

- Maya Angelou

"Hope is a state of mind, not a state of the world."

- Václav Havel

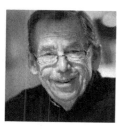

3

TABLE OF CONTENTS

Introduction

I know what you're think-
ing...this little fellow must
have had a wonderful
childhood. Unfortunately, the
opposite was true. But, to
avoid the use of trigger
words, suffice it to say that I
was born highly sensitive into
an insensitive family. Life was
unnecessarily painful and
melodramatic, and I left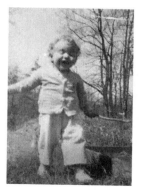
home as soon as possible after my 16th birthday.

I was fortunate to meet the love of my life at 18 and, showing a totally lapse in judgment, she married me soon after. Even though we're happily together these many (55) years later, I wouldn't recommend young people take this path. I guess one might say ours is a cautionary tale!

Meanwhile, I was able to become the kind of husband and father that I never had. And defied expectations by having a successful career in information technology and wrote several books including *Romancing the Buddha (3rd edition)*, *My Fifty Years of Buddhist Practice,* and *Personal Growth in the Time of COVID.*

Of particular relevance to this book is that I experienced many of the challenges today's teenagers (and adults) are facing. And while I lack a certain degree of maturity, my (74) years of age have afforded me a wealth of lessons learned.

For the last eight years, I've imparted some of this hard-earned wisdom to all the local ninth graders.

And, in this book, I've tried as honestly and concisely as possible to answer eleven of the more pressing questions teenagers have shared with me.

I'm grateful to Bainbridge Youth Services for sponsoring my initial high school presentations and hope this small book helps teens and their parents or guardians navigate what can be difficult but very rewarding years.

Note: All the illustrations were generated using artificial intelligence web applications and then further manipulated in Adobe Photoshop.

What is most important in life?

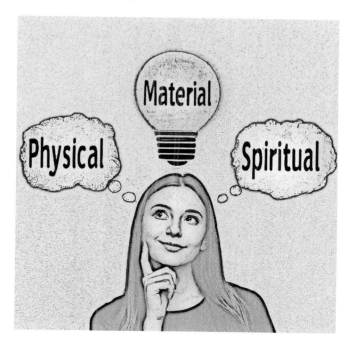

Without wisdom, inner resolve, and compassion for yourself and others, your physical and material accomplishments will lack meaning.

As a young adult, it might appear that you can only be happy if you get outstanding grades, attend the best school, have perfect health, the ideal job, and the partner of your dreams. While all these material and physical "treasures" (see next figure) are desirable, it is the nature of our attachment to them that can become problematic.

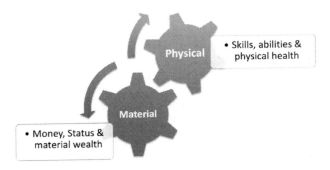

I have an affinity for psychological studies that are finding more and more that people in their fifties and sixties whose primary focus in life was the attainment of 'extrinsic goals' - externals such as wealth, property, fame, and status - tend to experience a higher level of anxiety, suffer more from illness, and have less sense of fulfillment.

It has been suggested that positive psychological constructs such as life satisfaction, positive affect, purpose/meaning, and optimism are generally predictive of better physical health and functioning.

So, while pursuing physical and material happiness, it is equally important when you're young to grow spiritually -- to develop treasures of the heart (see next figure) -- the ability to make wise decisions, the courage to never give up, and compassion for yourself and others. These attributes will give real meaning to all your external endeavors and accomplishments.

The importance of these treasures of the heart became very clear to me in the fall of 1971 when I took the bullet train from Tokyo to Nara Prefecture where I attended an afternoon discussion meeting

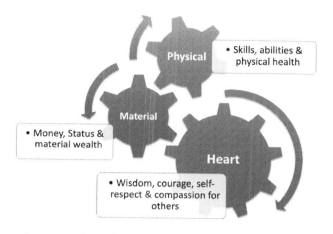

Physical
• Skills, abilities & physical health

Material
• Money, Status & material wealth

Heart
• Wisdom, courage, self-respect & compassion for others

and spent the night at the home of an architect. Unfortunately, I don't recall my host's name, so I'm going to call him Hiroshi because it means generous in Kanji.

Around 7 p.m., Hiroshi apologized that dinner was so late because his wife and mother-in-law had yet to return from a memorial service in Osaka. Sitting directly across from me, speaking through a local translator, he told me the story of the lady whose funeral his wife was attending.

During the atomic bomb in Nagasaki, this woman lost her husband and four young children. While many people might have succumbed to despair, she

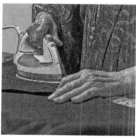 proceeded to adopt four war orphans, two boys and two girls. For the next 25 years, she sewed dresses and suits as well as mended clothes to earn enough money to feed and send her children to school. Hiroshi explained

that all four had excellent jobs and two were married with their own children.

He wanted me to know that this lady was the type of person who never turned away someone in need. She once even answered a middle-of-the-night knock on her door to repair a tear in his coat for a business trip he was taking the next morning.

Hiroshi's wife and her mother returned a few hours later exhausted from their journey. It turned out that several hundred people who knew this amazing lady had come out to honor her at the memorial service. Only after everyone had offered a traditional stick of incense and shared stories were they able to take the train home.

At this point, Hiroshi excused himself and went to another room and returned with something small in his grasp. He reverently placed a gold-plated tie clasp with an inset diamond in my hand.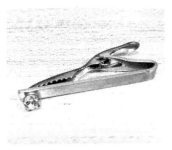

I remember his exact words. *"This is my most valuable possession that was given to me by my father. I see in your eyes that you are still discovering who you want to be in this life. Please remember this lady who mended so many lives whenever you lose your way. Ask yourself, could anyone have lived a more noble and admirable life than her? Let this be your guide whenever you're feeling lost."*

I almost didn't need the translator, so penetrating were his words. Tears flowed down my face. I wore that tie clasp for many years as a reminder of the importance of continuing to develop the spiritual aspect of my life.

Of course, the efforts I made to build financial security and take care of my health were important. However, I'm glad I placed the most value on developing wisdom, inner resolve, and compassion for myself and others. Without these, the physical and material results would have lacked meaning.

Each of you will need to find your own unique spiritual path. It might be your family religion, meditation, yoga, running, journaling, therapy, self-help books, or volunteering to name just a few. Ultimately, prioritizing personal growth and emotional intelligence will lead to a more fulfilling and meaningful life.

What if I don't know who I want to be?

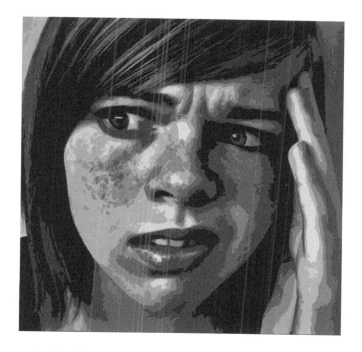

Anxiety happens when you think you have to figure out everything today.

Some of you may have strong feelings about the direction you want to go from a professional perspective. Or, you may have no idea at all!

My brother knew from a young age that he wanted to be a dentist. He doggedly pursued and achieved his goal. Now that he is retired, he provides free dental care to children all over the world.

Meanwhile, my parents wanted me to be an optometrist even though I had no interest in it. Upon (barely) graduating high school, I lived in in my car and, occasionally, on a friend's couch. I had absolutely no idea what the next day was going to bring much less my future career.

I eventually graduated college and have lived a surprisingly rich productive work life filled with many obstacles and victories and, most important, no regret. But my career gradually evolved as opposed to being planned. The lesson 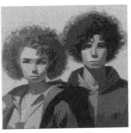 here is that both my brother and I ended up with rewarding professions even though we followed completely different paths.

My two daughters (a journalism professor and an attorney) ended up having careers that greatly differed from their interest in science in high school and college.

You may have peers who know what they want to do but there is absolutely no need for you to worry. Uncertainty about your future is not a weakness. Many adults grapple with the same thing. Your sincere efforts to do your best in the tasks before you will be the cause for future growth. It's better to give yourself time to explore than to force yourself to make a premature decision.

Here are five other things to keep in mind:

Be open-minded. Use this period of uncertainty as a chance to explore different interests, hobbies, and subjects. Try new things, take diverse classes, volunteer, or intern in various fields. You might discover a passion you never knew you had. Sometimes the best path forward isn't always the most obvious one.

Be patient. It's okay not to have everything figured out. Give yourself the time and space to explore and learn about yourself. Remember that your interests and goals may evolve over time, and that's perfectly normal.

Solicit advice. Don't hesitate to reach out to trusted adults, mentors, therapists, or career counselors for guidance. They can offer valuable insights and resources to help you clarify your interests and goals.

Trust the process. As long as you're actively exploring and learning, you're moving in the right direction. Trust yourself to make decisions that align with your values and aspirations.

And for those of you who know what job you want to pursue, allow yourself to take some different school electives and participate in extra-curricular activities. You might discover new interests and you'll be more able to relate to a broader range of people...something that will help you succeed later in life.

Meanwhile, take your time! Life is a marathon, not a sprint.

What if I struggle with depression?

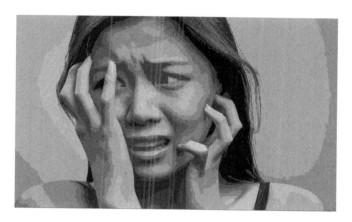

You are not alone and you are not broken!

I feel your pain. I spent most of my teens in the 1960s extremely depressed, took too many drugs, stole to buy them, and was unable to function at school. I kept losing jobs, hung out with equally dysfunctional friends, and had little interest in living. Sadly, back then no one talked about depression, antidepressants, or psychotherapy.

In my late teens, I hit rock bottom and was desperate to change my life. I was lucky, through a quirk of hippie fate, to have my wife and then a daily spiritual practice enter my life.

Still, it wasn't until I was in my forties, when my wife got multiple sclerosis (MS) and had to learn how to walk again, that my emotional bathtub overflowed. I finally realized I had to talk to a therapist and take medicine while I worked on getting better. With this help, I was able to regain my emotional equilibrium and experience a much happier daily life.

Some key actions I wish I could have taken when I was a teenager include:

Reach out for support. Opening up about your struggles can be difficult, but sharing your feelings with someone who cares, such as a therapist or physician, can provide immense relief and help you feel less alone.

Prioritize self-care. Make self-care a priority in your daily routine. This includes getting enough sleep, eating nutritious meals, exercising regularly, and engaging in activities that bring you joy and relaxation. Taking care of your physical and emotional well-being is crucial for managing depression and anxiety.

Practice mindfulness and relaxation. Explore mindfulness meditation, deep breathing exercises, or progressive muscle relaxation to help calm your mind and alleviate symptoms of anxiety. These techniques can help you stay grounded in the present moment and reduce overwhelming worries and stress.

Challenge negative thoughts. Learn to question the negative thoughts and beliefs that contribute to your depression and anxiety. Replace them with more realistic and positive perspectives. A professional trained in cognitive-behavioral therapy (CBT) can be particularly helpful in identifying and changing harmful thinking patterns.

Set realistic goals. Break tasks into smaller, manageable steps and set realistic goals for yourself. Celebrate your achievements, no matter how small, and be compassionate with yourself when things don't go as planned.

Remember that healing takes time. Recovery from depression and anxiety is a journey, and it's okay to progress at your own pace. I'm living proof that with time, support, and perseverance, you can handle these emotional challenges and lead a fulfilling life.

Above all, seeking help is a sign of strength, not weakness. You deserve to receive the care and support you need to navigate through this difficult period in your life.

What if my friend has depression?

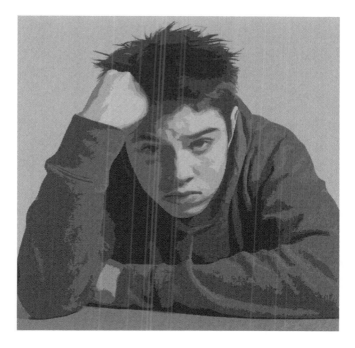

One of the most important things you can do is to let people know they are not alone.

None of your friends wake up in the morning hoping they have diabetes. It's not something they get to choose. And if your friend comes to school feeling really lethargic because they didn't take their insulin, you'll probably encourage them to go home and take it.

Having depression is no different. And neither is taking medication to treat it. If feeling down or anxious isn't something you have to deal with, you might be tempted to wonder why your friend with depression doesn't "snap out of it." But, believe me, we would if we could!

So, please don't judge your friends who are in the midst of an emotional crisis. They need your support. One way a high school student can help a friend with depression is by simply being there for them. Listening to their feelings without judgment and offering a shoulder to lean on can make a world of difference. It's important to let your friend know that you care about them and that you are there to support them through their struggles.

Encouraging your friend to seek professional help is another important step in helping them cope with depression. This could involve suggesting therapy or counseling services, or even accompanying them to their appointments for moral support. It's essential to remind your friend that it's okay to ask for help and that seeking treatment is a sign of strength, not weakness.

Additionally, engaging in activities that your friend enjoys can help lift their spirits and provide a temporary distraction from their negative thoughts. Whether it's going for a walk, watching a movie, or simply spending time together, showing your friend that you are there to share moments of joy with them can have a positive impact on their mental well-being.

It's important to educate yourself about depression and its symptoms so that you can better understand what your friend is going through. By learning about the condition, you can offer more informed support and help your friend navigate their feelings in a healthy way.

However, don't feel like you have to solve their problems. You aren't expected to have all the answers. And don't forget to take care of yourself, too.

On the other hand, it won't always be obvious that someone is struggling. Several years ago, a few students made some negative comments on Instagram about the unusual clothes a fellow teen had worn to school. No one knew that this young lady was feeling emotionally overwhelmed with her personal demons and the state of the world. Reading the online posts really upset her. And the students who posted those comments on social media felt badly when they found out. It doesn't take much to constitute bullying.

So, let's avoid judging others, treat everyone with respect, and lend a supportive hand to those in need.

What if I get a bad grade?

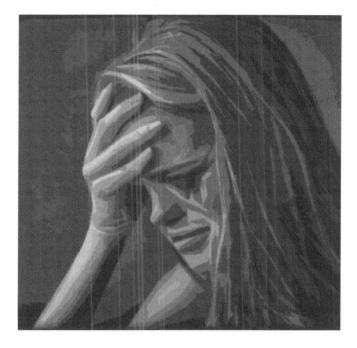

Strive for continuous improvement, instead of perfection.

Grades are a useful measure of scholastic achievement. But you are much more than your grades!

The pitfalls of striving for perfection can lead to burnout, anxiety, and a negative impact on your overall well-being. It's important to find a balance between academic success and self-care. Remember to take breaks, engage in activities you enjoy, and prioritize your mental health.

Of course, trying to get straight A's is a wonderful goal. But, so is doing your very best and getting straight B's!

There is a popular saying, "You can't spend your neighbor's wealth." So, don't waste time comparing with others. Be happy for your friend's accomplishments. Their success in no way diminishes your worth since the only person you can be is you. And no matter how hard you try you can't be them.

One of the first steps you can take after receiving a bad grade is to reflect on what went wrong. Did you not study enough? Were you struggling with the material? By identifying the root cause of the bad grade, you can take steps to address it and prevent it from happening again in the future.

It's also important for you to seek help when needed. Whether it's talking to your teacher for clarification on the material, seeking tutoring, or forming study groups with classmates, there are plenty of resources available to help you improve your grades.

Setting high goals, especially while you're young, is a smart thing to do. However, keep in mind that expecting perfection is futile!

What if I make a mistake?

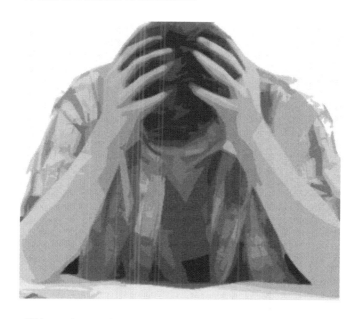

"I hope that in this year to come, you make mistakes. Because if you are making mistakes, then you are making new things, trying new things, learning, living, pushing yourself, changing yourself, changing your world. You're doing things you've never done before, and more importantly, you're doing something."
- Neil Gaiman

One of the biggest concerns expressed by our local high school students in an online survey I conducted was that they berated themselves when they made a mistake.

In 1976, I was the co-organizer of the City of New York's Bicentennial parade. My friend and I did a great job of delegating responsibilities, but at the last minute I decided that only I was capable of leading the several convertible sports cars carrying the VIPs including the governor to the review stand. Unfortunately, I hadn't taken the time to remind myself of the parade route, so I guided the waving VIPs past the review stand and almost all the way to Central Park! After turning the cars around, I had to part several marching bands, drill teams, and horseback riders to get the VIPs back to where they belonged. Truly a chaotic experience for all involved. However, I learned a valuable lesson about checking every detail of a plan, trusting others to fulfill their tasks, and the negative impact of arrogance.

Of course, when you make a mistake, you will probably feel a combination of emotions including vulnerability, regret, dismay, and guilt. These reactions are normal. The challenge is to find the lesson in the mistake -- like discovering new capabilities or how to be more patient with yourself and others.

So, stop belittling yourself when you do something wrong or disappoint someone. After all, mistakes are how you learn what does and doesn't work. It's a crucial aspect of development.

Admit your mistake before someone else exaggerates the story. Once you've self-reflected on your behavior and, if necessary, apologized, move on. Don't make things worse by reminding everyone how sorry you are. Dwelling on your failure only lends it greater import. Instead, make a new determination and proceed to grow by making even more mistakes!

To quote author Steve Goodier, *"Bring it up, make amends, forgive yourself. It sounds simple, but don't think for a second that it is easy. Getting free from the tyranny of past mistakes can be hard work, but definitely worth the effort. And the payoff is health, wholeness, and inner peace. In other words, you get your life back."*

I recently learned about a Japanese art form known as Kentsugi. This is a method of repairing cracked pottery by mending the broken areas with lacquer dusted or 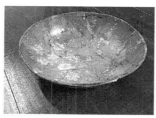 mixed with powdered gold, silver, or platinum. The underlying philosophy is that breakage and repair is part of the history of an object and need not be hidden. What a great metaphor for healing the metaphysical cracks we carry around. It means many of our weaknesses and habits are a thing of beauty -- a reminder of life's imperfections and the importance of humility.

How can I improve my relationships?

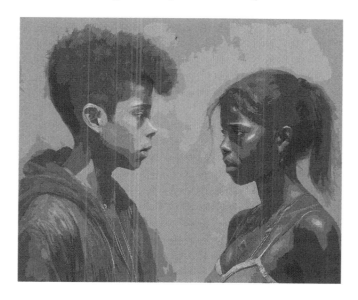

We live in the midst of a flood of soulless information. And the more we rely on one-way communication...the more I feel the need to stress the value of the sound of the human voice. The simple but precious interaction of voice and voice, person and person, the exchange of life with life." - Daisaku Ikeda

There was a time in the 1990s, when no matter how hard I tried, I couldn't get along with one of my work colleagues, who I'll call, "Bob." Bob had a way of getting under everyone's skin -- especially through the tone of his emails. My 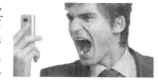 responses, which seemed so innocent and compassionate at the time, only made him more antagonistic.

I reflected a lot about this relationship and received encouragement from a trusted friend. She had me close my eyes and imagine that I was someone else talking to my coworker – a person I really admired for their compassion and wisdom. Instead of firing off a quick email response to yet another angry message that had landed in my inbox, I imagined this person walking from my office down to Bob's and, using a very warm voice, asking him how he was doing. I realized right away that this was the kind of caring attitude I needed to manifest.

The very next day, Bob and I ended up waiting for a government official in a conference room. I asked him how his family was doing. He said his teenage daughter had been diagnosed with diabetes a year before and had been refusing to take her insulin treatments. This was causing their family a lot of stress. I mentioned to him that it was a very difficult time for me because my wife of many years had recently been diagnosed with multiple sclerosis. Through this heart-to-heart sharing, Bob and I went from a relationship built on distrust to one of mutual respect. I've never forgotten this experience.

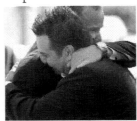

I read somewhere that about ten percent of our communications is what we say, forty percent is the way we say it (rate, tone, and inflection), and fifty percent is our body language before, during, and after we say it. So, what we write to each other needs to be extremely concise to be correctly understood. Written communication is missing the crucial sounds of a human voice and the visual context clues that show what the sender was actually feeling and whether the recipient was greatly upset, mildly peeved, or encouraged. It often takes person-to-person dialogue to grasp someone's true intention and to improve a negative situation. It is one of the ways we can create harmony in our surroundings.

When you feel compelled to write an emotional e-mail or text, first send it to yourself and reread it the next day before forwarding it to anyone else. By taking time to reflect, you can ask yourself if it would be more effective to just call the source of your frustration rather than slinging a one-sided written message. Such emotional barbs are impossible to recall and can cause considerable damage. How can you know if the recipient really understood what you meant if you can't see or at least talk to that person?

Here are few other tips:

Work well with others. Whether at school or at work, teamwork is often the key to success. If you're on a ship, the fact that the hole is on the other side is little consolation.

Be reliable and trustworthy. It's important to follow through on your commitments, be honest and dependable. By demonstrating reliability and trust-worthiness, you can build strong and lasting relationships.

Respect others. Gossip and negativity create disunity, reflect poorly on our own character, and drain our energy when we need it the most. There will always be something to complain about. Instead, express appreciation and recognize other people's strengths.

Support your teacher or supervisor. When we least want to talk to our teacher or boss is the most important time to knock on his or her door. It is the individuals we dislike that we can often learn the most from by engaging in honest dialogue. Don't run from adversity.

Don't always have to be right. Fellow students or co-workers who disagree with you aren't necessarily stupid. Other people want to succeed, too. Their values and perspective might just differ from yours. There isn't always a right and wrong way. Seek to understand other people's point of view and find win-win solutions.

Communicate clearly. Finally, if you're a great listener, try to express yourself more often. How else will other people get to learn who you are? But, if like me, you tend to be the one who does most of the talking, work on becoming a more active listener.

How important is balance in my life?

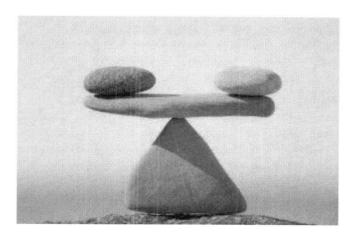

In the end, it's all a question of balance.

Finding a good balance in life is crucial for students as they navigate through their academic, social, and personal responsibilities. Volunteering for activities can provide you with valuable experiences, opportunities for personal growth, and a chance to give back to your community. It can also help you develop important skills such as leadership, teamwork, and time management. However, it is important to recognize when you're taking on too much and need to say no. Taking on too many commitments can lead to stress, burnout, and a decline in academic performance. In the long run, it will impact your mental and physical health.

It's important to prioritize your well-being and learn to set boundaries when necessary. This means being able to assess your current workload, commitments, and personal needs before agreeing to take on additional responsibilities. By learning to say no, you can avoid spreading yourself too thin and focus on activities that truly align with your goals and interests.

Some people overcommit even when it jeopardizes their mental and physical health. In my twenties, when I tried to slow down, I would be overcome with dark feelings. So, I tried to "stay afloat" by saying yes to everything and filling my schedule. Eventually, I crashed.

Through all of this turmoil, an excellent therapist and a supportive family enabled me to develop the wisdom to survive and even flourish. I learned that I didn't have to do everything -- that I could say no. It was quite a relief.

A critical first step is to realize that your environmental situation will often manifest your state of mind. So, if your thoughts are clouded, you will be like a tarnished mirror that reflects the negativity around you. But, when polished, you can become like a clear mirror that reflects the more positive aspects of your reality. The trick is to regularly do some activity to polish your inner mirror in whatever form best fits you.

As a young manager at an aerospace company in the 1980s, my peers were working very long hours. Just for curiosity's sake, I asked different executives if there was anything in their career that they would have done differently if given the chance. Their answers gave me a lot to think about.

Every single one told me that they wished they hadn't worked such long hours and that, in hindsight, they should have avoided bringing their work home. As a result, many of them ended up divorced and estranged from their adult children. I made a strong determination to make my relationship with my wife and daughters a priority. With business travel and regular deadlines, maintaining a work-family balance was always on my mind. I once flew home to Virginia from Amsterdam just to catch one of my daughter's ballet recitals and then took a plane back to London the next day. She never forgot that. I also made it a habit to leave the office on time unless I had critical work to get done as opposed to just staying late because others were. There are many excellent articles on the Internet about how to say no. But the first step is to grasp why it is important to sometimes take a pass. This one change can revolutionize your life. It's the difference between being overwhelmed and feeling in control. Learning how to prioritize takes discipline but is a critical habit to develop while you're younger.

What risks should I take?

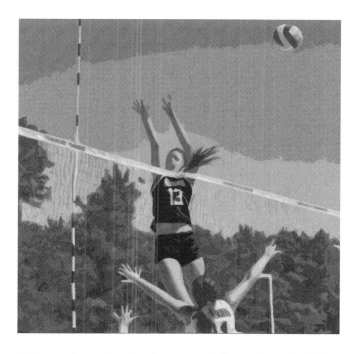

"If you always do what is easy and choose the path of least resistance, you never step outside your comfort zone. Great things don't come from comfort zones." – Roy Bennett

The benefits of going out of your comfort zone can be immense. By taking positive risks, you can develop new skills and gain valuable experiences that will build confidence and self-esteem as you learn to overcome challenges.

Because you no longer spend most of your time with your parents or guardian, you are definitely an independent young adult. As such, you are responsible for the consequences of the actions you take. This means you need to make wise decisions regarding substance abuse, reckless driving, and bullying. These actions can have serious consequences, both short and long term. For example, substance abuse can lead to addiction, health problems, and legal issues, while reckless driving can 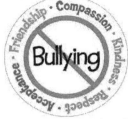 result in accidents, injuries, and death. Bullying can have lasting negative effects on both the victim and the perpetrator, impacting their mental health and relationships.

I learned the hard way that the negative causes I made in high school trained my brain to need an external chemical stimulus to manage my moods. It took many years of therapy and a strong spiritual practice to learn how to manifest joy from within my life.

When I look back, I can see that every single meaningful experience in my life was a direct result of some action I took. And these usually involved some degree of risk. Whether it was running away with my girlfriend in 1969 (which I don't necessarily recommend!), moving from California to Virginia with our family in 1984, and then to Bainbridge Island in 2004, or starting my own consulting business in 1999, it seems that whenever I ventured out of my comfort zone, my life improved. This is a life lesson I'm glad to share with you!

Can I make a difference in the world?

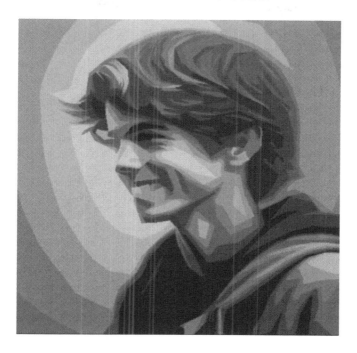

"The best way to not feel hopeless is to get up and do something. Don't wait for good things to happen to you. If you go out and make some good things happen, you will fill the world with hope, you will fill yourself with hope."
- *Barack Obama*

Many people are feeling overwhelmed by today's uncertain social and political realities -- feeling powerless about their ability to make a difference. I recall experiencing a similar despair in the 1960s. I have vivid memories of the school bell ringing three times to alert us to drop beneath our desks in case of an atomic bomb attack. Coupled with the war in

Viet Nam and the absence of civil rights for a large segment of our population, there seemed to be little reason to have hope for the future.

There has never been a time in modern human history without conflict, injustice, and suffering. But there has also never been a time without compassion, resistance, and relief. There has been and perhaps will always be the potential for both darkness and enlightenment. And the world will always reflect this dichotomy and the resulting tension.

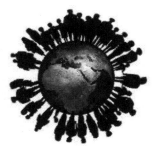

The fact there are over eight billion people in the world can make us feel insignificant. What do we matter and how can we possibly make a difference? But each of us is unique. There is no other person exactly like us in the entire universe! We each get to create our own story unlike anyone else's. The only question we need to answer is how we can be our best possible selves in the time we have.

In a fascinating paper in the 2017 International Journal of Wellbeing, psychologist Ashley Buchanan proposes bringing together two areas of research -- a "being well" perspective from positive psychology and a socially and ecologically orientated "doing good" perspective.

He gives the example of benefit mindset as everyday leaders who seek to "be well" and "do good." Wouldn't that be refreshing?

Eight years ago, I challenged the ninth graders at our local high school to befriend just one person during the school year who they perhaps wouldn't normally associate with. After one of my talks, I watched as one of the students, who I'll call Alice, probably figuring she would get it over with as soon as possible, walked up to a girl we'll call Mary after class. A few months later, the health teacher told me Alice was shocked to learn that Mary had been living

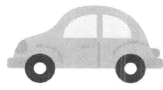

in a car with her mother at a local park. They were hiding from her abusive alcoholic father. Because Alice took the time to ask her a few questions, Mary decided to try harder at her new school and began making friends. Four years later, she graduated with excellent grades. And this year she will be completing an undergraduate degree at the University of Washington.

So, clearly Alice made a difference!

Buddhist scholar Daisaku Ikeda has said, *"When we change, the world changes. The key to all change is in our inner transformation -- a change of our hearts and minds. This is human revolution. We all have the power to change. When we realize this truth, we can bring forth that power anywhere, anytime, and in any situation."*

Each of us has the ability to impact the world in significant ways. After all, if a flapping butterfly wing can cause major changes on the other side of the world, surely our efforts for peace and justice can counter the fundamental darkness we have all been experiencing.

I believe that the best course of action is to pursue a path of inner change and to manifest the resulting compassion and wisdom as action towards peace in the world around us. Every single person you come in contact with is important. This truth gives me confidence that each of us can build a happier life and make a positive difference in the world.

How can I feel hopeful?

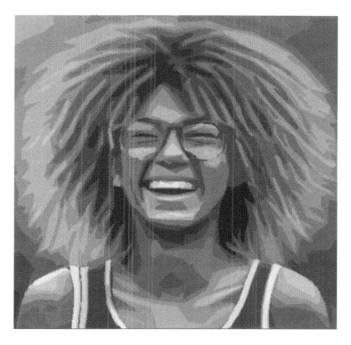

"When hope has eluded me and I can see nothing but the pain within which I sit, I remember that a horizon cannot exist without two sides; the one I can see and the one that I cannot." - Craig D. Lounsbrough.

I recall driving with my family in an overheated four-door Chevy with no seat belts across a barren Texas desert to begin a new life in Los Angeles. It was the summer of 1961, the year the Berlin Wall was built, Freedom Riders took buses into the South to bravely challenge segregation, and the top song was "Will You Love Me Tomorrow' by the Shirelles, a question I keep asking my wife to this day.

While dodging my father's vigorous backhand in another futile attempt to stop my brother and me from bickering, I noticed that no matter how far we traveled, we never seemed to reach the horizon. Even though I knew we lived on a revolving sphere, it still seemed mysterious.

Speaking of seemingly unattainable horizons, my wife recently reminisced how confident we were in the late sixties that our acts of civil unrest would result in an end to global conflict, hunger, and racial injustice. Life turned out to be a harsher reality as if someone kept moving the goal line.

"The wideness of the horizon has to be inside us, cannot be anywhere but inside us, otherwise what we speak about is geographic distances." - Ella Maillart

Fortunately, we encountered a spiritual practice that values even the smallest efforts of kindness towards ourselves and others regardless of the socio-economic and political state of affairs. This implies an acceptance that the creation of a truly harmonious human race, something that is beyond our immediate grasp, is more a journey than a destination. Each day presents us with the choice of what impact our thoughts, words and actions will have on the world around us. This is a difficult but essential truth if we are to contribute to the ongoing evolution of our species over the next thousand years.

I admit that it's easier to accept the theoretical validity of this perspective than to put it into practice. Especially with those whose behavior or attitude I find objectionable. I can only imagine how difficult this is for you, the next generation, who must grapple with so many personal and global threats. But therein lies the challenge that each of us faces every day for as long we're alive. To quote J.R.R. Tolkien, *"There is some good in this world, and it's worth fighting for."*

Remember that, as Václav Havel said, *"Hope comes from your mind, not the state of the world."* This means that while it's natural to feel discouraged when you're experiencing hardship or loss, you don't have to remain in that condition. Avoid hanging around cynical people. And when you're having negative thoughts yourself, seek out someone who can raise your spirits.

It may seem trite, but you'll be grateful later in life if you take the time now to work on your personal growth in whatever constructive ways fit you best. This will pay huge dividends in the future!

Self-assessment questions

Here are some self-assessment questions you can revisit every month or so to identify any areas needing improvement.

Are you:

- Dreaming Big?
- Accepting life's uncertainty?
- Getting help when you need it?
- Avoiding comparing yourself to others?
- Learning from mistakes & not beating yourself up?
- Keeping activities in balance (saying no, when necessary)?
- Taking steps to be more hopeful about life, school & world events?
- Going out of your comfort zone?
- Trying to make a difference?
- Making informed & wise decisions?
- Listening with an open mind?
- Treating yourself & others with respect & compassion?

Made in the USA
Columbia, SC
22 May 2024